HowExpert

CW00539977

Herbali

How to Grow Herbs, Learn
About Holistic Health, and
Become a Herbalist From A to Z

HowExpert with Heather Phelos

Copyright HowExpert™
www.HowExpert.com

**For more tips related to this
topic, visit
HowExpert.com/herbalism.**

Recommended Resources

- HowExpert.com – Quick 'How To' Guides on All Topics by Everyday Experts.
- HowExpert.com/books – HowExpert Books
- HowExpert.com/products – HowExpert Products
- HowExpert.com/courses – HowExpert Courses
- HowExpert.com/clothing – HowExpert Clothing
- HowExpert.com/membership – Learn All Topics from A to Z by Real Experts.
- HowExpert.com/affiliates – HowExpert Affiliate Program
- HowExpert.com/jobs – HowExpert Jobs
- HowExpert.com/writers – Write About Your #1 Passion/Knowledge/Expertise.
- YouTube.com/HowExpert – Subscribe to HowExpert YouTube.
- Instagram.com/HowExpert – Follow HowExpert on Instagram.
- Facebook.com/HowExpert – Follow HowExpert on Facebook.

Table of Contents

Prologue:

Holism is harmony and balance in mind, body, and spirit which ensures a high quality of life, calm and sound mind, high efficiency in cells, happiness, and continual thriving.

We look far and wide for an outside source to tell us how to live and what to eat. Interestingly, the more we look, the further we are to hearing the truth of the matter. It takes looking inward, testing the health-waters, and experimenting in real life to understand what is best for our bodies. Some practices may work for one person's body chemistry but not for our own. We are extremely complex and unique beings and even the most acclaimed research cannot tell you what is best for your own body. The path to wholeness is different for everybody. That being said, research and ancient wisdoms give us a jumping off point for our journey to begin.

The study of herbal medicine usage has been in every culture for millennia, as a solution to just about every ailment. Plants and herbs are our allies to a healthy lifestyle and they infuse universal and ancient wisdom into our daily lives. The study and subsequent practice of herbalism can be an invaluable tool in taking control of your health and becoming closer to the biodynamics of earth.

The goal for this book is to begin a journey to becoming holistically health- minded through herbalism. That is, using herbs as an ally to not only create balance, harmony, and peace within our mind, body, and soul but to do so ethically and sustainable for the earth, as well. Herbalism is not just a physical practice but a meditation and connection to the pantheism of nature. It is a part of a dynamic health, one that incorporates moving parts and philosophies to optimize our living and happiness through individual relationship with your herbs.

Key points for reading this book:

- Plant medicine and herbalism are used interchangeably in this book because the whole of the plant (root, flowers, leaves, bark), as well as fruits, nuts, and vegetables are recommended in the practice. Fungi is also addressed in this book.
- Herbs are multi-dimensional and as infinite in possibilities as humans. You nor I will ever know *everything* about a plant. They often have dozens of known characteristics so don't get discouraged if herbal studies make you feel overwhelmed!
- This book is a strong skeleton for herbalism but it by no means encompasses everything, it is meant to be used as a guide for your own future studies! There are literally thousands of herbs worldwide so herbalism can be a lifelong study. This book is set up as a framework to begin your journey into herbalism: from understanding your herbs, their history, and chemistry to planting and harvesting.

- To begin your herbalism journey, I urge you to keep a journal on how your herbs grow and how your body interacts with different herbs.

<u>Disclaimer</u>: Your health is your own responsibility, as with any treatment course whether allopathic or holistic, you should do your own research and/or consult with medical professionals to ensure this fits into your goals and values.

Chapter 1: An Overview to Herbalism

This chapter serves as a thorough introduction to the various spheres of herbalism: the history and cultural contexts, and how the practice can improve your life.

What is Herbalism?

If you think back far enough, you probably remember yourself picking off a honeysuckle from its bush, pulling out the long stem, and drinking the single drop of honey that each flower holds. Or maybe you remember taking a bite of a tangy wood sorrel clover found in your lawn or perhaps dodging the large, tough, and pungent bay leaf in your mom's homemade chicken soup? If you have experienced mingling with the plant world, to some degree, you have experienced the art of herbalism.

DID YOU KNOW

HERBALISM IS THE POTENT PRECURSOR TO MANY PRESCRIPTION AND OVER-THE-COUNTER DRUGS. FOR INSTANCE, WILLOW BARK IS THE ACTIVE INGREDIENT IN ASPIRIN

Herbalism is the foundation of the whole of medicine: both ancient and modern. It is the study of using herbs medicinally, either by ingesting, smoking, or applying topically.

Herbalism History

As the OG Medicine of the world, traditional herbalism is the most ancient, yet living tradition in the world. These medicines transverse *thousands* of years and withstand the test of time, now if that isn't evidence- based, I don't know what is!

From the beginning…

Around 3 billion years ago, plants and humans shared the same common ancestor [1]. These similarities are reflected in our DNA, giving us the ability to interact and live symbiotically.

Known herbal usage started in Paleolithic graves and cave drawings over 60,000 years ago and within the oral tradition of herbal shamanism in Asia and South America over 30,000 years ago [2]. From the dawn of humanity, we know that humans have been utilizing native herbs as nutrition when foraging or gathering.

'But when did humans discover medicinal uses for herbs?' One might ask. Some of the first writings *ever* were about the medicinal qualities of herbs. Over 5500 years ago, Mesopotamia became the birth place of urban areas, cuneiform writing, and known medicinal herbalism [2]! For the years following, the world quickly followed suit. Herbal writings appeared in India, China, and Africa in the 3rd millennia B.C. Soon thereafter, the famous Greek physician, Hippocrates, set the wheel of herbalism and modern medicine in motion. He wrote about how food and plants should be treated like medicine and was living proof for this philosophy because he lived to be 90 years old [3]! Herbalism boomed in the Renaissance (along with many other art forms) and remained the main form of medicine for the next 500 years, although there were some dips during the Witch Trials [4]. Nicholas Culpepper was instrumental in organizing contemporary herbalism of the 1600's, so much so that his work is still used today. It was not until the rise of the American Medical Association in 1920, that herbalism began to decline [4].

Snapshot of herbalism writing:

Cuneiform Clay Tablets	Pen Tsao	Rig Vedas	Ebers Papyrus	Hippocrates	Dioscorides De Materia Medica	Monk Physicians	Canon of Medicine-Hakim	Various authors/ Herbal boom
Mesopotamia	China	India	Egypt	Greece	Rome	Europe	Unani tradition	Europe
3500 BC	3000-2800 BC	3000-2500 BC	1500 Bc	~400 BC	79 AD	Middle Ages	1000 AD	1400-on

International Snapshot- A peak through the cultural lenses of Herbalism

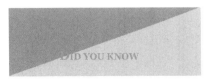

Herbalism is a worldwide practice. In the following chapters, we will unpack the herbalist cultures of Traditional Chinese, Ayurveda (or Traditional Indian Medicine), various African, South American and Latin American, Native American, and European medicines. There is some overlap in medicine (as expected) when cultures and countries are on the same continent. For instance, in TCM and Ayurveda, about half of the plant sources overlap. Since the spice trade and other forms of globalization, herbalism expanded to more universal terms.

Some of the world's herbalism practices were diminished by colonialism, cultural imperialism, toxic rulership, and exploitation of native lands and peoples. The Midwives and medicine women of Europe were burned at the stake during Witch Trials of the 16th and 17th century. Native Americans decimated to a mere 1% after colonization. The slave trade in Africa uprooted communities at a time to a foreign land. *Diminished*, but not *extinguished*.

Modern place in society

Unfortunately, in today's society, herbs are not as widely used and revered. Herbalism in western civilization is more of a fringe, or alternative art rather than infused into daily life. As allopathic medicine moved into the forefront in the 20th century, herbalism and other "alternative" therapies were pushed aside. Many remedies were transformed from their natural herbal forms, so you may be surprised of the herbal knowledge you already have in your pocket. For instance, Ginger Ale is often given for stomach aches. Ginger is a potent digestive aid and anti-inflammatory herb. Echinacea and honey are often advertised in cough drops as an immunity booster or sore throat reliever.

Recently, there is an herbal revivalist movement due to the increasing costs and side effects of prescription drugs, antibiotic resistances, and lack of relief or cure for chronic disease. Traditional and plant medicine is resurging in popularity all over the world.

Traditional medicine needs support in *all* countries.

In upper-income countries:

Herbalism can aid in treating insidious and under-researched chronic diseases such as Lyme's, or serve as a healing connection to nature that our minimal down-time, high-stress society craves. Herbalism is key to holistic health and is extremely important in this urban, unnatural world we live in today. It is the missing link to just plain "eating healthy and exercising," and can aid in nourishment, endurance, and vigor. Not only can the practice help us succeed in our physical, mental, or spiritual goals but it can help us thrive and go above and beyond.

In low to middle income countries:

As well as all the reasons stated above, herbalism is extremely important for the wellbeing of the people. For many cultures in Africa, traditional medicine was always at the forefront of healing, due to distrust in western medicine or lack of hospital access. Herbalism holds a deep and ancestral link and keeps tradition and culture alive.

For some areas in China, Traditional Medicine is used in adjunction to allopathic medicine, and it is an integral part of the national health programs. Despite the known efficacy of traditional medicine in Chinese and Indian clinical trials, much of herbalism in western cultures remains on the fringe. I believe it is due to a lack of government funding on herbal studies within the States and a distrust in herbal efficacy:

Herbalism is still associated with a type of "magical" or "witchy" sphere and less of a science, despite research that proves differently.

We often still use imagery and language associated with herbs, showing our deep and interwoven relationship and co-inhabitance with the plant world. For instance, the metaphor of "Sage Advice" is used for wise and knowledgeable advice through someone who has experienced and lived the truth. Sage has long been revered as an herb for elders, as it supposedly helps remembrance and enhance insightfulness. An olive branch has been the symbol of peace for thousands of years. And lastly, plants and humans have the same personality characteristics: bitter, sweet, cold, warm, salty (retaining emotions, resentment like salts retain water).

From the Sacred to the Mundane

LIFE HACK

CITRONELLA IS A POTENT MOSQUITO REPELLANT.
BONUS: PREVENTATIVE FOR THE DEADLIEST ANIMAL ON THE PLANET
BONUS #2: TRADITIONAL MOSQUITO REPELLANTS ARE LOADED WITH CHEMICALS

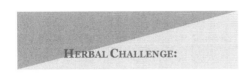

Herbalism has many purposes and places within a
given society. It is one of those practices that presents
itself differently with every question you ask and
dependent on the purpose of your practice. Herbalism
generally focuses on medicine but can be used in
beauty regimens, aromatics, spiritual rituals,
vitamins, and flavoring. Medicinally speaking,
herbalism can be used allopathically, which is
reactionary, or seeks to fix an acute problem. It can be
used in chronic disease or pain management which
requires a more dynamic approach, or it can be used
as preventative medicine or aiding to optimize health.
These approaches can be intertwined and require
knowledge on herbal actions and interactions. It is
important to start a relationship with the herbs you
work with in order to understand their needs in
growing and to understand how your body chemistry
interacts with the herbs. This can be researched
through plant diets.

Medicinal Purposes

Herbalism can treat both infectious and chronic
diseases, or be used as a preventative.

HEATHER'S SUN INFUSED OIL

INFUSE LAVENDER + CALENDULA IN A CARRIER OIL OVER 4 WEEKS IN THE SUN. ADD VITAMIN E FOR PRESERVATION AND FOR AN EXTRA SKIN BOOST. THIS TRIPLES AS A SKIN CALMER & CLEARER, MOISTURIZER, SUN PROTECTANT, AND GIVES OFF A NICE SCENT

Many dishes utilize herbs to flavor their foods or for aesthetics. Think about all the herbs you use on a weekly basis: Herbs De Provence (savory, thyme, basil, marjoram, lavender, parsley, oregano, tarragon, rosemary, fennel seed, and bay powder from the South of France) to flavor your chicken. Oregano and basil to top your favorite Italian pasta dish. Indian Masala Chai spiced with cinnamon, clove, and cardamom. Chili powder to bring a kick to your Latin American dishes. You can even add edible flowers to your dishes. Chances are you have seen a fruit tray with lovely purple orchids strewn about; well this flower is just as nourishing as the fruit it sits upon. Most likely you have been receiving the medicinal and nutritional aspects of herbs well before you knew. There's nothing wrong with utilizing the herb for its flavor (I encourage you to let herbs ignite your senses!) but these herbs are way more multi-dimensional and powerful than we may initially believe.

Fragrance

I challenge you to take a look at the products you are using. Do any of them have the generic ingredient of "Fragrance" in it? The term is basically a mask for any and all chemicals a company would like to throw into a product. It is conveniently masked under this term and can include mild irritants to severe carcinogenic, endocrine disruptors, and toxins. This lack of transparency is a huge problem. The Environmental Working Group labels Fragrance as an 8/10 in toxicity – or a "high concern" [5]. Instead there are plenty of other ways to get the scent you prefer in addition to reaping the benefits of the aromatic medicinal qualities of essential oils and herbal blends. You can smoke an herb by directly burning herbs in a fire-safe dish, or place it in a dish above a candle with a carrier oil. If you would like to make a scented lotion, try sun infused oils with your favorite aromatic herb.

Become Inquisitive of Your Products and Ingredients:

I urge you to consider going straight to the source of these remedies rather than the branded versions which are often extremely diluted, filled with sugar, or chemically changed- all which affect the health and potency of the herb.

Let's take a look at the ingredients in store-bought Aloe sun burn relief and the health and environment implications:

Banana Boat Aloe Lotion: Water, SD Alcohol 40, Glycerin, Polysorbate 20, Carbomer, Triethanolamine, Imidazolidinyl Urea, Aloe Barbadensis Leaf Juice, Fragrance, Iodopropynyl Butylcarbamate, Benzophenone-4, Yellow 5, Blue 1.

As you can see, Aloe is the eighth ingredient in a store-bought aloe gel. Rather than going straight to the source of an Aloe Vera plant, you have twelve other ingredients including dyes and semi-toxic materials. Where the plant can be ingested or applied topically, store-bought gels are absolutely toxic. A good rule of thumb is if you cannot pronounce the ingredients, you should probably stay away from it. If your products look more like a chemistry project straight from a lab, the product is most likely riddled with toxins that are harmful to our cells and DNA. To find out more about the toxicity of

ingredients in your products, EWG.org is a wonderful resource.

DID YOU KNOW

BASIL HAS SIMILAR COMPOUNDS (I.E. VERY ANTI-INFLAMMATORY) AS MEDICAL CANNABIS BUT WITHOUT THE HIGH. IT HAS BEEN A RELIGIOUS HERB FOR OVER 4,000 YEARS, WITH HOLDS IN RELIGIONS SUCH AS HINDUISM, ORTHODOX, AND JUDAISM.

Nutrients

Herbs are chock full of nutrients. They are extremely bioavailable to our cells and way more so than ingesting commercial vitamins. Packaged vitamins are minimally effective due to synthetic ingredients. Also, herbs can increase the bioavailability of other herbs and foods, called a bioavailable enhancer.

Rituals

Herbs are used in a variety of spiritual contexts. You may even find some amazing historical uses for the herbs in your own garden! I encourage you to research the religious history of your favorite herbs.

Included is a <u>short</u> list of various herbal ritual uses:

- Sage Smudging to dispel negative energy
- Master plant teachers (entheogens) or psychedelics for spiritual journeys and shamanism
- Palo Santo burning to create sacred space
- floral baths to recharge and revitalize during full moons
- Pipe smoke of Mugwort used as an oneirogen, or herb that induce dreams

Why get into herbalism?

As stated above, herbalism is a way to get back to our roots and the source of potent medicine that our ancestors have used for millennia before us. Herbalism can help us be self-sufficient instead of relying on store-bought products that are filled with toxins. Through self-reliance, we have control of what we put in our bodies and can save tons of money by relinquishing our tight bond with consumerism. Through biodynamics, herbalism can help save our environment by reducing plastic and waste and by cleaning and purifying the quality of our soil and air. Biodynamic herbalism creates a relationship between humanity and the environment. In addition, herbalism is a stepping stone to living our optimal life and creates a foundation for other healthy choices. It can heal our woes from disease to mental fog and disturbances to skin conditions and much more. Herbalism can aid in spirituality, helping us connect to old earth traditions and in conjunction with rituals. And best of all, herbalism is easy, free to start, and it is fun helping life to grow!

It is easy to start

Go to a local farmer's market or home improvement store and pick up a few starter plants. Virtually every geographical location is capable of growing their own plants and herbs. Minimal knowledge is needed to get started but plant wisdom will continue to unfold the more you work with plants.

It helps the planet

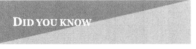

DID YOU KNOW

HERBAL BOUQUETS WERE MADE POPULAR BECAUSE
THE BELIEF THAT PLANTS HELD THE "LANGUAGE OF
LOVE." PLANTS SYMBOLIZED DIFFERENT MARITAL
BLESSINGS THROUGHOUT MANY ANCIENT CULTURES

By relying on yourself, you rely less on transportation of goods which in turn, lessens the amount of unnecessary travel pollution. Also, plants cancel out carbon admissions! While practicing sustainable herbalism, you utilize the resources in the environment, such as rain water and natural soil to fuel your plants. Composting ensures there is less daily output of waste and in turn, less landfill debris. Gardening also helps wildlife preservation by adding to the health of the ecosystem and provides food for the bees and worms which are essential! Also, herbalism helps the soil and air quality by creating more biodiversity. Your environment becomes cleaner and in turn, purifies itself. It regenerates new life and heals past pollutions [6]. Indoor plants, such as Aloe and Ivy can help purify and improve indoor air quality by acting as potent cleansers in the removal of VOCs (pollutants that caused hole in ozone so just imagine what they can do to our bodies!) [6].

It helps us connect to the earth

The best medicine is one that you have a part in every step of the way. One that you can breathe life and intention in. One that you know where the plant came from and know it was planted, grown, harvested, and turned into medicine by you. Studies show that this form of medicine is way more potent. Respectful plant medicine-making which involves symbiotically living with nature, is just as important as the herb in healing!

It promotes self-reliance

And less reliance on consumerism. Self- grown herbs ensure the best taste and quality. Commercial herbs are often picked before nutritional maturity, could be sprayed with chemicals, grown in a non- biodynamic way (monoculture and mass producing- similar to the way the health of livestock decline when raised only for profit), artificially enhanced (coloring, GMOs), may have been picked years ago and no longer potent. This self- reliance also saves money. Commercial herbs can be extremely overpriced. There is no comparison between an herb that is a one-time cost of $2 on average for seeds (or free, if you are in a seed sharing community) to ~$10 per 100g bottle.

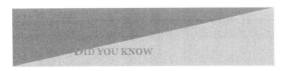

DID YOU KNOW

MISTLETOE HAS BEEN ASSOCIATED WITH DECEMBER FESTIVITIES FOR OVER 3000 YEARS. THE MYSTICAL PROPERTIES BELIEVED TO BE IN MISTLETOE WERE ADOPTED BY CHRISTIANITY FOR CHRISTMASTIME FROM OTHER PRE-CHRISTIAN RELIGIONS SUCH AS NORDIC YULE

It aids holistic health

Not only can herbalism be used to heal virtually any problem but the act of gardening shows healing effects too! Through plants, you can get nutrition, make all your beauty and skincare products by hand, and flavor your food. Herbalism also aids in mental health, sleeping, dreaming, healing, and can boost energy, longevity, and your immune system.

24

Herbalism can be used as a fragrance or by aromatherapy.

Aid to spirituality

Ancestors have been using herbs in rituals for millennia. Herbs and human history are as connected as humans pondering their purpose and creator, so naturally, the three are inextricably linked.

Herbalism can be used in conjunction with rituals and spirituality. There is a reason why every religion utilizes herbs during prayer. In Christianity, two out of the three gifts to Jesus were herbs. Frankincense symbolizes the divine spirit, due to the smoking of incense, and Myrrh was used as embalming oil so it was a symbol to the mortality of Jesus. In Hinduism, sedative herbs are burned as incense in the temples during prayer. Holy Basil (Tulsi) is revered as a sacred healing Goddess itself since the Vedic Times (beginning in 1500 BC) [7]. Similar practices can be found in Islam and Judaism. In Anglo-Saxan Paganism, there were 9 sacred herbs: Mugwort, plantain, chamomile, watercress, nettle, crab apple, french parsley, and fennel [7]. Herbs can be used to cleanse the spirit and mind, and prepare us for meditation or prayer to bring us closer to the divine.

Wildcrafting, foraging, biodynamics, and permaculture principles

These are all forms of taking a holistic, ecological, and balanced approach to herbalism. Wildcrafting is a form of foraging within a plant's natural habitat. Unused plants can be utilized and this promotes new growth. In this manner, the plants are in their most whole and natural form. This can be used as an adjunct to growing in your own sustainable ways. Biodynamics and permaculture takes this a step further and brings nature into the homestead. It entails creating a harmonious plant and animal ecosystem that is sustainable and contributes to the health of each component. Biodynamics include but is not limited to: composting your food scraps, crop rotation, biodiverse planting, rain collection, and working with good bacteria.

Why it's one of the most potent medicine

These principles ensure that your practice is optimal for the surrounding ecosystem and in turn, ensures optimal nutrition. Biodynamics and wildcrafting incorporate the most natural form of growth and merriment with nature and surrounding environments which creates the most potent form of medicines.

How to do so safely

Be able to recognize plants with confidence by smell,
look, growth habits, and knowing what similar plants
look like so you can avoid foraging those instead! Use
apps such as Picture This to help identify plants.

Ethical considerations

Do so responsibly and humanely: do not take more
than you need. There is a delicate plant ecosystem
that you should be considerate of. Also, be aware of
endangered plants. If you should stumble upon an
endangered plant, you should *protect* it rather than
harvesting.

Chapter 2: Understanding your Herbs

To fully understand your herbs, you will need to take a deeper look into the background and purposes of your herbs. Monographs will typically give a snapshot of the herb in providing information such as the scientific name, herbal family, geographic region, medicinal parts, herbal actions, uses, and recommended dosage. Dependent on the length of your monograph, you may need to do a bit more research for historical and spiritual uses. Delving into the background of your herbs will take your herbalism practice a step further. Herbalism is partly an anthropologic lens into our ancestors' lives. Worldwide, our ancestors relied heavily on the medicine of herbs. This research can connect us to deeper meanings and wisdoms, ground us to our pasts, and help us understand our place in the world.

 This historical and geographical lens will start to bring pieces of the herb puzzle together.

Geographic and culture herbal origin

Traditional Chinese Herbs

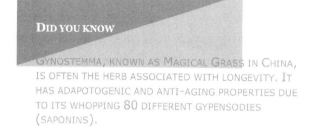

DID YOU KNOW

GYNOSTEMMA, KNOWN AS MAGICAL GRASS IN CHINA, IS OFTEN THE HERB ASSOCIATED WITH LONGEVITY. IT HAS ADAPOTOGENIC AND ANTI-AGING PROPERTIES DUE TO ITS WHOPPING 80 DIFFERENT GYPENSODIES (SAPONINS).

TCM is a patient-centered form of medicine. It is based on the principles of balancing yin, yang, and the five elements while promoting vital life force energy (Qi) and healthy function of the 12 meridians [8]. It prescribes physical exercise and meditation in addition to plant and animal medicines. The focus is on harmony and treating disease symptoms holistically. Spotlight herbs in TCM include the following:

Ginseng, Reishi Mushrooms, Motherwort, Licorice, He Shoe Wu, Angelica, ashwagandha, schisandra berries, Eleuthero, Gingko Biloba, Goji berries, Rhodiola Succulent (especially potent when combined with Schisandra berries), Gynostemma, and White Peony.

White Peony Monograph:

History: Peonies have been used for millennia in China, once revered for its beauty, quickly became medicinal in purpose.

In the middle ages, Europeans thought of peonies as symbols for femininity, love, abundance, and a happy union. Medicinally, peonies treated pain of childbirth, headaches, and asthma. Peonies celebrate a 12th wedding anniversary and can survive for a century, growing perennially.

Medicinal usage: aids in detoxification, enhances healthy hair and skin, reduces pain induced by chronic illnesses and menstrual cramps, balances immune system, and relieves insomnia and anxiety.

Ayurveda

Ayurveda is very similar to TCM in that is it patient-centered, holistic, and focuses on harmony within the body for optimal health [9]. It is based on the principles of balancing elements, in particular: bodily constitutions called Doshas, which regulate every physiological and psychological process in the living organism [9]. Spotlight herbs in Ayurveda include the following:

Bitter melon, Black pepper, Fenugreek, Holy basil (Tulsi), Clove, Cardamom, and Turmeric

Turmeric Monograph:

Used for over 4000 years in India as a medicinal and sacred herb, Turmeric has over 25 names in Sanskrit, often referring to its luckiness, deep color, medicinal properties, or divine symbolism [9].

Medicinal purposes include arthritis treatment, GI and menstrual cramp disturbances reduction, blood purification, improves blood circulation, and treats skin conditions [9].

Properties: bioactive compound curcumin, anti-inflammatory, anti-cancer, antimicrobial, carminative, and anti- phlegmatic

Native American medicine

Native American Medicine is very earth-centered [10]. Although there may be some tribal differences, plant medicine is infused in every sphere: biological, social, spiritual, and ritual, as well as the arts of healing mind and body [10]. Many tribes believe in pantheism, or that everything has a spirit and is interconnected [10]. The plants are a part of the community. For United States herbalist, these plants will be the most native:

Catnip, Elderberry, Goldenrod, Sarsaparilla, Red clover, Skullcap, Black Cohosh, Bee Balm, Echinacea, and Raspberry Leaf

Bee Balm Monograph:

Also, known as Monarda or Bergamot tribes used the flowers for sweat baths at the sign of an illness. They also bathed their infants in Monarda water [10].

Medicinal usage: relieves sore throats, fevers, bronchial illnesses, depression, gastrointestinal disturbances, and for menstrual cramps.

Echinacea Monograph:

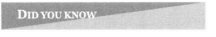

DID YOU KNOW

MINT IS FOUND ON NEARLY EVERY CONTINENT

Native healers would use the plant (nicknamed Snakeroot) for wounds, snake bites, and respiratory infections [10]. In the 1870's, Dr. Meyers patented Echinacea in "Meyer's Blood Purifier" as a cure for all ailments, in particular- infectious diseases [11].

Medicinal usage: fights infection in the body, heals yeast infections and torn connective tissue.

Properties: immune-stimulant, antibiotic against staphylococcus and Streptococcus, bactericidal, lymphatic tonic, cytokine against tumors, and collagen protectant [11].

Raspberry Leaf Monograph:

History: Mainly used as "womb medicine," that is, to relieve heavy and painful menstrual cycles and to provide relief for morning sickness and laboring [12]. Red Raspberry Leaf is supposed to prevent miscarriages and create a fertile womb space.

Folklore: Echinacea makes women extra fertile if tea is dosed in a waxing moon phase.

Research: Published in Aust Coll Midwives Inc Journal. in 1999, "women who ingest raspberry leaf might be less likely to receive an artificial rupture of their membranes, or require a caesarean section, forceps or vacuum birth than the women in the control group" [12].

European Medicine

European Herbalism was made popular by Hippocrates and used by countless ancient philosophers and physicians such as Pliny the Elder. It is used throughout history for the past 2000 years. Spotlight herbs in Traditional European Medicine include the following:

Chamomile, Witch hazel, Sage, Hops, Feverfew, Evening primrose, Belladonna, Woodruff, Valerian, calendula, lemon balm, rosemary, and St. John's Wort.

Lemon Balm Monograph:

HISTORY OF CALENDULA:
LATIN FOR CALENDAR, BECAUSE IT WAS OBSERVED THAT
THE FLOWERS BLOOMED AT THE FIRST OF EVERY MONTH.
- USED AS A BEAUTY TREATMENT BY ANCIENT
  EGYPTIANS
- WORN AT WEDDINGS IN MODERN AND ANCIENT
  INDIA
- IN MEXICO, CALENDULA ADORNS THE ALTARS
  DURING THE DAY OF THE DEAD

Used in the Mediterranean for over 2000 years as a
'calming' herb and a longevity agent. Also, used at the
temple of Artemis as a sacred herb [13]. Carmelite
water (also known as the 'Spirit of Melissa') was used
all over Europe in the Renaissance age as a nervous
tonic and as perfume water for hair and skin [13].

Medicinal usage: Sleep and digestive aid, reduces
anxiety, mosquito repellant, prevents tumors, reduces

34

negative effects of Alzheimer's Disease, softens wrinkles, boosts alertness, sharpens memory, and supports liver detox [13].

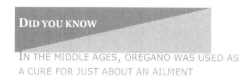

Rosemary Monograph:

Rosemary's Latin name means dew from the sea because its origin was near the Mediterranean Sea [14]. Rosemary is a very hearty and stable herb.

History: Ancient Egyptians, Greeks, and Romans thought of Rosemary as an herb to remember the dead [14]. It has been used in herbalism and symbolism for over 2500 years. Anne of Cleves gave sprigs of Rosemary to every guest at her wedding with Henry the 8th [14]. Many of the first printed herbalism books (ranging from 1515-1590) mentioned Rosemary for its antioxidant properties, gout relief, and plaque protection [14].

Medicinal usage: Insect repellant, improves brain function, aids digestion, improves circulation, hair growth, liver detoxification, reduces stress, balances hormones, and prevents blood clots.

Properties: bitter astringent, antioxidant, vitamin B6, calcium, iron, antiseptic, vitamin c, antifungal, antiulcer, anticancer, and anti- phlegmatic.

Times for use: Vitamin, topical hair, and skin care.

"Grow for two ends…Be it for my bridal, or my burial" – Robert Herrick on the diverse symbolism of Rosemary [14].

St. John's Wort Monograph:

Origins: Mediterranean, Greece

It is associated with St. John because it blooms near his feast day and because it is said to bleed red in olive oil near the date of St. John's beheading (August 29) [15].

Medicinal usage: Depression, wound healing, and pain reliever for menstrual cramps.

Properties: analgesic, antibacterial, antiviral, antioxidant, neuroprotector, and antinociceptive [15].

Times for use: Monthly moon, mental disorder, and wound poultice.

New research shows St. John's Wort effectiveness in reducing Opium dependence [15].

South American/ Latin American

South American herbalism is one of the oldest medicines. Shamans worked with plants for tens of thousands of millennia in prehistory, or before writing began. Many of these traditions still exist today. The rich Amazon Rainforest is home to the most potent and nutrient rich plants, such as Maca and Cacao. Latin American Medicine was a combination of Spanish colonization, South American natives, and African traditions from the Slave Trade. Spotlight herbs in the South and Central Americas include the following:

Maca, Yerba Matte, Plantain leaf, Coca Leaves, Cacao, Soursop, Acai, Cayenne, Irish Sea Moss Red Algae

African

This broad category encompasses: Northern: Egyptian, Moroccan, Unani/ Arabic, South and Central African Medicines. African traditional medicine is imbued in African traditional culture and holds with it much ritual importance, as well as supporting National health where allopathic hospitals fail. Spotlight herbs in the continent of Africa include the following:

Honeybush, Wormwood, Devil's Claw, Gotu kola, Rooibos, Gum Arabic, Aloe Vera

Aloe Vera

Monograph:

Aloe has been used on every continent for thousands of years and is known as the plant of immortality and the "wand of heaven" [16]. It has been used for health and beauty for over 6,000 years in Egypt [16]. It has over 200 bioactive ingredients including a plethora of vitamins and minerals. It has Vitamin B12, which is uncommon for plants. It boasts collagen stimulating properties and boosts and the immune system [16]. It also acts a vitamin bioavailability enhancer. It has 20/22 essential amino acids [16]. A form known as Bitter Aloe is used throughout South Africa. Aloe can cure virtually any skin condition. It can also be used as a digestive stimulant. It also protects the skin from UV damage and treats sunburn. Cleopatra used Aloe religiously (double meaning of both in religiously ceremony and in the context of using Aloe every day) [16].

Chapter 3: Herbalism- A Science.

A scientific approach should be used in conjunction with purpose- driven research. A biological and chemical approach to understanding your herbs includes knowledge on herbal actions, constituents, tissue states, and organs associated.

Self-initiated herbalism includes recognizing, and seeking to balance, any disharmony in the body, therefore, aiding in holistic health. This is done through understanding the actions your herbs have on your body and choosing herbs that have adaptogenic, nutritive, and revitalizing effects.

Where to look for your purpose

For specific diseases or ailments, it is helpful to research herbal actions, or how herbs work in the body. Once you get a base knowledge, it may be wise to start a plant diet so you can see how these herbs work on you as an individual. Your body chemistry may require a slightly different dosage or an herbal combination to work potently. Your herbalism journal is imperative to this process.

If your purpose is holistic health, you may want to research the vitamin, antioxidant, and mineral components to your herbs. Herbs are some of the most nutrient dense foods on the planet.

By Treatment

Anatomy chart and most commonly associated herbs:

Brain and memory: peppermint, sage, turmeric, rosemary, thyme, gingko biloba, ginger

Nervous system: lavender, chamomile, astragalus, ashwagandha

Respiratory system: oregano, peppermint , osha, licorice, marshmallow, eucalyptus, elecampane

Skin: aloe, chamomile, tea tree, calendula, tamanu, lemon, honey

Kidney: dandelion, red clover, goldenrod, celery root, parsley, gynostemma

GI: fennel, peppermint, chamomile, lemon balm, licorice, kombucha (herbs + probiotics)

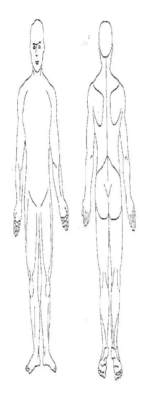

Hair: aloe, hibiscus, lavender, rose, green tea, nettles, rosemary, ginseng

Teeth: Echinacea, peppermint, sage

Eye: Fennel, golden seal, gingko, wolfberries

Heart: nettles, cinnamon, ginger, rosemary, garlic, rose, hibiscus, turmeric, hawthorn, motherwort, marjoram, woodruff

Reproductive: yarrow horny goat, red clover, black cohosh, saw palmetto, maca

Collagen: He Sho Wu, gynostemma, horsetail, nettles, comfrey, aloe

Gallbladder/ Liver: Milk thistle, green tea, marshmallow, beetroot

Herb actions, a simplistic guide

Diuretic promotes urination and excretion of water

Tonic revitalizes whole body

Stimulant enhances energy

Aromatics- promote respiratory or reproductive function and are the basis of aromatherapy (due to volatile oils)

Bitters- promote digestion

Mucilagins- aid in hydration and nutrition and coat mucous membranes

Adaptogen are some of the hottest topics today. These actions balance stress hormones by regulating the HPA (Hypothalamic Pituitary and Endocrine Axis). In turn, they boost energy, mood, metabolism, sex drive, immune system, and skin. Basically, everything a human could want in an herb! Many of these herbs also have highly nutritious content, lower inflammation, and fight free radicals. These are the quintessential "holism" herbs [17].

Alterative restore proper function of body

Astringent causes closing or contraction

Nervine calms the nerves

Expectorant promotes secretions in lungs and throat

beauty purposes

Herbal concoctions can be used in place of all unnatural beauty products. Not only can you cleanse, clear, moisturize, and correct skin and hair imbalances but they can also be made up into make-up products. Herbal concoctions are ingested or applied topically for beauty enhancements.

Through Preventative measures

If you are just simply aiding in holistic health, look to nutritive blends. Research the vitamin, mineral, and antioxidant material in the plants. You can also consider the plant energetics to address any imbalances you feel before they turn into disease.

Active constituents are the parts of the plant that yield a medicinal effect. The main 16 categories are: Alkanoids, Anthocyanins, Anthraquinones, Bitter, Cardiac Glycosides, Coumarins, Cyanogenic

Glycosides, Flavanoids, Glucosilinates, Minerals, Mucilage, Phenols, Saponins, Tannins, Vitamins, Volatile Oils [17]. There are 13 essential vitamins and 16 essential minerals. Plants are abundant in all but K2 (which can be found in fermented foods), B12 (which can be found in Nori Seaweed & Aloe), and D3 (which you can get from the sun)!

Nutrient dense Plants as vitamins:

 Seaweed Garlic, green tea, ginger, turmeric, basil, cilantro, pepper/spearmint, tarragon, oregano, thyme, parsley, dill, and chives

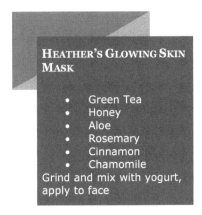

HEATHER'S GLOWING SKIN MASK

- Green Tea
- Honey
- Aloe
- Rosemary
- Cinnamon
- Chamomile

Grind and mix with yogurt, apply to face

By taste

Pungent herbs can be spicy, acrid, or aromatic. They promote whole body organ function, act as a carminative, immunomodulator, and diaphoretic. Spicy herbs include garlic, cayenne, ginger, turmeric, horseradish, cumin, oregano. Acrid herbs upregulate the parasympathetic nervous system and promote relaxation. These herbs include valerian, catnip, hops, and Kava Kava. Aromatic herbs have a high

44

concentration of volatile oils. These herbs include Tulsi, peppermint, fennel, cardamom, and rosemary. Cinnamon is both sweet, aromatic, and spicy so it provides benefits from both and is a warming herb which is different from most sweet herbs.

Sweet herbs provide nourishment to our tissues and promote growth. They act as a blood tonifier and have actions in the pancreas, spleen, and stomach. They often have qualities of being mucilagionous, immunomodulation, and calming. Herbs that sweet include marshmallow, licorice, honey, slippery elm, astragalus, stevia, chamomile

Salty herbs are known for their high mineral content and diuretic qualities. These herbs include nettles, red clover, seaweeds.

Sour taste is often obtained through ingesting fermented foods or fruit acids. Sours provide us with antioxidants and minerals. They also aid digestion, promote healthy liver and gallbladder function, promote hydration, and remove excess heat from the body. Herbs that are included in this taste category are Schisandra, rosehips, raspberry leaf, wood sorrel, and hawthorn berries.

Bitter herbs are an extremely important taste for GI function but are often under- represented in Western diet. They are drying, astringent, and tonifying. They are known for their alkaloids and aid in detoxification. They are nervines and lymphagogues (promotes lymph function). Herbs in the bitter category include coffee beans, dandelion greens, yarrow, aloe, witch hazel. These herbs can provide tannins (red wine) and can act as mind altering substances: peyote, coca, ayahuasca, coca, poppy, tobacco.

Tissue states/ Energetics

The study of tissue state energetics is a link between imbalances and elements, which is globally studied in all traditional medicines. Transmuted into different cultures with varying names and components, the key philosophy holds the same: we need unique medicine to treat disharmony in a unique person. These patterns or constitutions are linked with our personality, metabolism, and physical structure and hold a feedback loop to signal imbalances. It takes self-inquiry to address disharmony before disease starts (preventatively) and within disease (treating symptoms, discovering cures). These imbalances can be broken down into tissue states:

Tissue states are patterns of imbalance addressed by herbalism, the three states each have two polarities [17].

Tissue state #1: **Tension**

<u>Dilation/ Relax</u>: tiredness or lack expression

Treat with astringents: Sumac, Rose, Witch Hazel

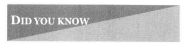

DID YOU KNOW ROASTED DANDELION ROOTS
CAN BE SUBSTITUTE FOR COFFEE, LESS
ACIDIC + MORE NUTRITIOUS

<u>Constriction/ tension</u>- overexcited muscles, adrenal dysfunction

Treat with acrid or bitter sedatives and nervines: lavender, valerian, hops, St. Johns Wort, Gotu Kola, milky oats, skullcap, motherwort, kava kava, and holy basil.

Tissue state #2: Rate of tissue function, heat

<u>Depression/ slow/ cold:</u> low function and necrosis

treat with warming volatile oils and adaptogens: cinnamon, ginseng, garlic, cayenne, basil, ginger, horseradish, and fire ciders (warming herbs with apple cider vinegars).

<u>Excitation/ fast/ hot:</u> too much heat, inflammation, redness, overactive immune responses, burn out, or auto- immune symptoms.

Treat with sour or mucilaginous, cooling herbs with adaptogens: tart flowery herbs such as rose, hibiscus, peach leaf, Marshmallow, ashwagandha, and schisandra berries.

Tissue state #3: Density/ moisture

<u>Torpor/Swollen/ damp:</u> Accumulation and putrefying of dead material.

Treat with alteratives and revitalizing herbs: Nettles, dandelion root, red clover, oatstraw, Ginseng, rosemary, tulsi, and rhodiola.

Or Astringent: yarrow, witch hazel, red raspberry

<u>Atrophy/brittle/dry:</u> Withering, aging tissue

Treat with sweet, nourishing herbs: comfrey, marshmallow, and healthy oils and fats.

HERB FAMILIES:
ARE A CLASSIFICATION BASED ON HERBS WITH
SIMILAR TASTE, CONSTITUENTS, AND VISUAL
CHARACTERISTICS - MOST CULINARY HERBS ARE
IN THE LAMIACEAE FAMILY (MINT FAMILY) THEY
ARE USUALLY AROMATIC. HERBS IN THIS FAMILY
INCLUDE:

Chapter 4: Action Plan for the Wise Herbalist

Medicine is most potent when it comes from a personal relationship. Planting, growing, and harvesting from yourself with love and gratitude will infuse happiness into the plant's and your own DNA. It is wise to do your research before getting into herbalism. No, you do not need to be a master herbalist before planting your first seed (which would be near impossible because you need to practice to become a master, anyway) but you should be familiar with your herbs preferences and uses. There is no magical recipe to beginning a relationship with your herbs but I suggest picking a purpose then learning about your herbs' backgrounds, growth patterns, and how they interact with human biology. Your herbal knowledge can and should grow within your journey but it is wise to be forward thinking, as well. You will want to make the most out of your harvest and ensure your craft will not spoil or go to waste. Consider ideas of preserving your harvests. And lastly, your action plan should have a sustainability component. Deadheaded parts can be used in a compost and turned into nutrients for new growth. It's the cycle of life, baby! There should be no waste in this process and a composted garden will ensure bioavailable nutrients in your soil.

Picking a Purpose:

The best way to start your journey is to reflect on the reason you want to get into herbalism. Is there are a specific purpose you would like to explore?

Maybe, you would like to create an apothecary for certain ailments you would like to soothe. Perhaps you are thinking about creating all of your own beauty and cleaning products. Or maybe you want to delve into holism a little deeper. Whatever your purpose, think of how herbs can help you achieve your goals and how you can responsibly grow as an herbalist. Remember, herbs are wild, and a part of nature, but we are also entering a partnership with these herbs so you want to plant wisely and kindly.

Learning Phase:

Once you choose a focus for your study, start researching the types of herbs that can help you in this focus. You have creative freedom to learn about your herbs' simple actions, go deeper into their science, or even go a step further into the herbs' cultural and spiritual context. Recognition is key to ensure a safe harvest. A tip is to start slow- with one to a small handful of herbs and really get to know their innerworkings. Choose your herbs then start researching how to obtain the seeds or starter plants. You should also research their growing requirements to make sure you can provide for the herb. During this phase, you can start considering the end product. How would you like to turn your herbs into herbal products? This requires some knowledge in how to best preserve your herbs potency, dependent on the purpose and the mode of use. You may need to start obtaining a muslin cloth for drying your herbs, bottles for preserving your herbs, alcohol to create tinctures, or paper bags to store your herbs.

Planting Season:

Now that you have a solid base to herbal backgrounds and interactions- you are ready to take this relationship further, at home and into your (garden) bed. It is time to lay down the roots in becoming an herbal practioner. By this time, you will have narrowed down herbs you would like to grow. You will now have to make sure your garden has the requirements necessary for your plant. Sometimes, you will not have the capabilities to grow an herb yourself due to geography or garden space limitations so you make consider buying dried herbs from a reputable and biodynamic source and that is still great! I believe it is important to try growing herbs yourself to truly get into the rhythms of herbalism. There are diverse garden types to fit any of your needs and every geographic region has their own native medicinal herbs.

Start by visualizing your garden. Once you have an idea of how you would like to plant, start to ready your space. This may mean obtaining gardening tools, pulling weeds, turning soil, and adding manure to make sure your soil is fertile for your plants to thrive in. Next, you will need to obtain your herbs. Seeds can require a little more research than just simply placing them into soil. Potted plants may go through a phase called transplant shock and will need some time to adjust to the new soil.

Going with the flow:

This is the time to let your herbs do their thing. Remember, herbs and humans are allies so give them room to grow but listen to their language- they will let you know when they need help or additional maintenance (more or less water, sun, soil, etc.).

Hearty Harvesting:

Paying attention to your herbs will ensure a strong harvest. Some herbs need to be pruned and deadheaded so they can focus on new growth. Each herb has a different way of letting you know when it is time to harvest. During this time, you may choose to start creating your herbal remedies.

Sustainability:

A wise herbalist thinks of the past, present, and future of the herbs. They consider the growing patterns and how to last winters with minimal production. They also consider saving seeds for the next planting season and seeks to give back to the earth as gratitude.

Considerations before planting and growing your herbs:

Is the plant a Perennial, Biennial, or Annual?

Perennials lifetime tend to vary greatly from four years to a human lifetime. There flowering season is typically shorter, lasting just a few weeks. Some of my favorite perennials: lavender, sage, mint, lemon balm, thyme, oregano, and rosemary

Biennials take two years to complete their life cycle. In the second year, the plant flowers (to propagate) and then dies. These are sometimes self-seeders so they can be mistaken for perennials. Great biennials are parsley, mullein, and stevia. Advice when growing Stevia: Stevia can be used as a sweetener; it is said to be 50-200 times sweeter than sugar so use sparingly.

Annuals have one year in their life cycle but can be a self-seeding annual. German Chamomile is an annual flowering herb, unlike its perennial counterpart: Roman Chamomile, though it will self-seed. My German Chamomile hops into different spots in my palette garden every year. Other common annual herbs are dill, basil, and marjoram.

You will need to take note of your garden's components. Your herbs and garden should match in sun, space, and soil requirements. Consider placing your garden in an area that is away from pollution and easy to visit every day.

How much sun does the plant need?

Full Sun [6+ hours of direct sunlight]: most culinary herbs

Shade [0-3 hours of direct sunlight]: These plants can do well indoors and include mint, lemongrass (although mine grows rampantly outdoors in full sun), catnip, lemon balm, and thyme.

How much space does each plant need to grow?

Read up on the depth and spacing that each seed and eventual plant requires to thrive.

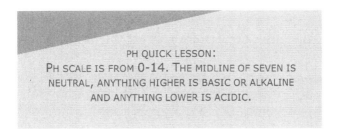

PH QUICK LESSON:
PH SCALE IS FROM 0-14. THE MIDLINE OF SEVEN IS NEUTRAL, ANYTHING HIGHER IS BASIC OR ALKALINE AND ANYTHING LOWER IS ACIDIC.

What type of soil does each plant need?

Types of soils include: fertilizer, manure, peat moss, planter's sand, rocks, potting soil, and composted nutrient rich soil. Acid loving plants include heathers, marigolds/ calendula, gardenia, dill, flowering trees, sweet potatoes, parsley, peppers, berries, and broccoli. Add sulfur, peat moss, and coffee grinds to make your soil more acidic. Basic loving plants include: yarrow, salvia, and lavender. Add lime, baking soda, or wood ashes to make your soil more basic. Neutral loving plants include: chives, ginger, mustard, and marjoram.

Drainage and aeration relates to how quickly your soil holds water and how much air can pass through your soil. Aeration is important because it allows nutrients, water, and oxygen to be more accessible to plants and their root systems. A healthy soil should be 25% air, 25% water, 40% mineral matter and 10% organic matter.

A well thought out planning phase will help ensure a smooth growing phase for your herbs; regardless, it is important to have a relationship with your plants. Understand the early signs of a distraught plant and how to troubleshoot with additional maintenance. Your plant may need some extra love and tenderness throughout its growing season so be attentive.

Troubleshooting:

Do your herbs continually soak in a puddle of water? Your soil may not be draining well enough or you may be overwatering your herbs

Is your leaves dead or dried out? You may be sun-burning the leaves if you water at the sun's highest point- try watering in the early morning and only water at the base of the plant. Are you watering enough? Are you deadheading enough so that nutrients go to just healthy growth?

Wilted: Is your plants seeing enough sunshine? Make sure your soil is full of nutrients by adding compost and manure.

How do I get my seeds ready for planting?

Scarification involves weakening, opening, or otherwise altering the coat of a seed to encourage germination. Stratifying or moisturizing seeds in a damp paper towel or seed starting in compostable egg crates is a great way to keep seeds indoor until they are strong enough to plant in outdoor settings.

Timing of seeding: a rule of thumb is hearty perennial herbs or cool season vegetables are to be planted in the fall, while annuals are to be planted in the spring.

DID YOU KNOW

FOR OVER 2000 YEARS, GREEKS AND ROMANS USED SAGE FOR SORCERY TO WARD OFF EVIL, TO INCREASE FERTILITY, AS A HEALING TONIC, AND AS A LOCAL ANESTHETIC. CELTIC DRUIDS SMOKED SAGE IN SACRED SPACES.

Garden types:

Palette gardens are a good way to ensure your plants are getting enough sunlight. Palette gardens are great for: patios or no access to ground, urban gardening, or gardeners low on pots. Palettes contain your herbs to a specific region. This is important for our versatile, hearty herbs such as lemon balm and mint which will take over a garden. Bonus: The soil in a palette garden is nutrient dense due to decomposition and living all in same area, it is harder for bugs and weeds to pop up, easier to maintain, and has the perfect drainage if you use a gardening mesh on the underside.

Indoor some herbs do great in container gardens and can be brought indoor for winter months. You can bring in most of your culinary herbs to a sun facing windowsill for winter. Succulents are great indoor plants. At first, I thought that succulents as a whole were mainly for decorations or ornamentals. Of course, I knew of agave and aloe as medicinal and culinary but that was about it. Boy, was I wrong! Succulents can be either ornamental or medicinal. Medicinal succulents include: Houseleek, Aloe, purslane, indian borage, Cuban oregano, rhodiola, jewels of opar, lechuguilla, prickly pear, sea asparagus, dragonfruit , and the list goes on and on! Some note on growing succulents: They like to be watered less frequently. In active months (April-November), water once per week. Let the soil get dry towards the end of the week. During dormancy, the winter months of November through March, water only once per month. Succulents like to have direct sunlight. P.S. all cacti are succulents but not all succulents are cacti!

Hydroponics This gardening does not use soil, just mineral infused water.

Sacred spirals and other shapes are used to maximize herbal growth and infuse ancient spiritualism into gardening. It is a way of raising herbs off the ground in order to create a small ecosystem of itself. These spirals may keep hydrophilic herbs close to the bottom (earthbound part) of the spiral. There are many garden designs that have ancient, spiritual, and logical context to them.

Hardiness zones

Hardiness zones are a reference guide for the climate in relation to plants that can survive here [18]. When researching your herbs, match their hardiness to the climate you live in.

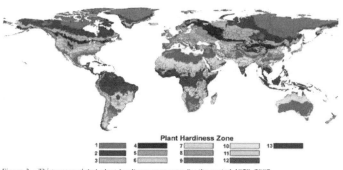

Plant Hardiness Zone

Figure 3 - Thirty-year global plant hardiness zone map for the period 1978–2007.

Placement of your herbs

Companion planting is a way of creating a symbiotic relationship between plants to aid in the health and in warding off diseases. This practice improves the health of the soil and plant alike. There is a whole science to companion planting but the universal plant companions are as follows: yarrow, stinging nettle, garlic, oregano, mint, basil, and tomatoes.

Chapter 5: Harvesting herbs

During the growing cycle, you will need to know the optimal time to harvest your plant. Each herb has a different way of letting you know when it is time to harvest. For instance, chamomile petals bend backwards when they are ready for harvest. This will ensure top potency and nutritional value. You will need to know how to pick your herbs. Some herbs prefer you cut at an angle (like roses), while others prefer you pick by hand an inch from the aerial parts. Some herbs may require root harvesting and others just leaves and flowers. Gather your herbs with respect and offer love, care, and gratitude back.

When to pick your herbs is **after** they have matured (which will be different for each herb). Maturity will ensure that your herb can keep growing (harvesting too much will be detrimental to your plant) and will ensure the best taste and nutritional value. But **before** flowering for peak nutrition and taste. Only harvest 1/3 of your plant at a time, harvesting too much will inhibit the ability to perform photosynthesis. The best time to harvest is in the morning, after the dew dries but before the strong heat of the day (between 8-10am).

How to pick your herbs: prune plants in a V manner for more yield: don't pick from the top. Cut dead/ dying/diseased parts for this will just start to weigh the whole plant down.

Chapter 6: Herbalism and Creation

This is where medicine-making takes place: using alchemy to transform raw plants into heightened abilities. The medicine you create will depend on the imbalance you are treating and the nutrients you want to preserve.

Fresh or dry

 First, you need to have the product in mind. Some medicines work better and more effectively with fresh herbs, others with dried. Before you harvest, have your materials ready. It isn't necessary to wash your herbs if you grow organically and pesticide free (and I urge you to do so!). Finer herbs are better fresh (like parsley), while hearty and thick herbs (like bay leaves) are better dried. Some herbs require drying for the medicinal properties to become more potent.

Dehydration techniques:

- Hang herbs upside down with cotton or burlap string- hang in dark, cool area
- Lay herbs on a flat muslin cloth and turn herbs over every few days
- Drying racks for aeration
- Quick dry via dehydrator, oven, or microwave – make sure herbs are set to very low heat

You will know herbs are well dried when they crumble easily. Tip: Before storing, all herbs must be completely dried or else they will be infected with mold! If dried properly, herbs will keep for ~6-12 months in full potency.

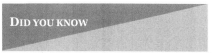

DID YOU KNOW

TO PREVENT STEAMING OFF VOLATILE OILS WHEN MAKING HOT INFUSIONS, KEEP TEA COVERED

Herbal Concoctions Table by Menstruum Type:

	Water	Alcohol	Oils	Apple Cider Vinegar
Preserves	sugars, proteins, gums, mucilaginous material, pectins, tannins, mineral salts, carbohydrates	Resins, alkaloids, glycosides, organic acids, chlorophyll, acrid/ bitter constituents	Aromatic, flavonoids, oils, alkamindes, resins	sugars, proteins, gums, pectins, tannins, mineral salts *mineral/ vitamin content, resins
Remedy Types	Cold infusion: nutritive, mucilaginous blends infused in cool water overnight Decoction: tougher parts of plants are simmered for over an hour to release benefits Hot Infusion- tea	Tinctures (must be 80+ proof)	Topical Essential oils Aromatherapy Healing Salve Sun Infused oils	Fire ciders Tinctures Great for tonic herbs or vitamin mixes

	can be mono or multi blended and steeped for up to 20 minutes			
	Flower essence- flowers soaked in water and sun infused for 4 hours			
Preservation length	3 days	5+ years	Up to 1 year	Up to 2 year

Miscellaneous: **Poultices** are herbs placed in a muslin cloth bundle, heated or moistened and applied to wounds.

Chapter 7: Sustainability

Sustainable gardening does not deplete the resources and environment. Rather, it adds to the diversity and health of an ecosystem. Follow these permaculture techniques to ensure sustainable living:

- If you are using annual herbs, look for seeding/self-sowing or make sure to save seeds
- Composting lowers waste and turns used material into new material in a beautiful cycle
- Use mulch to conserve water
- Diversify plants for cross pollination, pest control and to repel disease by promoting biodiversity
- Plant flowering herbs for bees
- Weed control via long hoe gardening and aerating soil. Learn to identify invasive plants and pull before they take charge
- Use your own organic pest control by companion planting
- Grow native herbs
- Crop rotate to make sure you are giving the land time to rejuvenate and to create soil biodiversity
- Used Vegetables scrapes can be turned into plants: keep stock/root in water, change often to avoid mold or bacteria buildup, and then plant roots down when they get larger and have some growth
- Winterize your perennials

Herbalism Seasonality

Herbalism interacts with the body and the environment. Our body's requirements and the herbs that are available differ depending on season.

> Winter: warming herbs, roots, immune tonics, fire ciders

> Summer: nutrition, hydration, cooling herbs, fruits

> Spring: reawaken, clearing, purifying, energy tonics

> Fall: hearty, end of season bounty and celebration

Post- Harvest checklist:

Before winter, it is time to prepare your garden for a long winter to ensure a bountiful spring

Harvest root systems for herbal needs   _____

only 1/3 so that you do not kill the next season's plants

Trim back old leaves so the roots can lie dormant

_____

Fully dry all herbs before labeling and stocking (name + harvest date)   _____

Supplement with ethical and biodynamic herbs if needed   _____

Be prepared for this to happen and do your research on a good provider beforehand

Pull all weeds and lay down mulch for warmth and spring weed control   _____

Bring in any herbs that can become seasonal indoor plants   _____

Communing with plants brings you closer to the natural world. A relationship with our plants means reciprocating the valuable medicine plants offer us by becoming guardians, plant warrior, and defender of nature. It is here that we think of ways to ensure sustainable and responsible practice.

Chapter 8: Summary and Plan of Action for Budding (pun intended) Herbalists!

Learn about your herbs

Scientific name, herbal family, folk name

Look and Recognition

Geography, history, and culture

Herbal Actions, Contraindications, and uses

Herb Constituents and Parts

Planting and growth patterns, timing, and requirements

Harvesting techniques

Companion plants and herbal pairings

Planning Phase

Start simple- Start with one to a handful of herbs and get to know them

Think space- What's your garden going to look like? How much sun will it get? What are native plants in your area?

Get tools- garden hoe, rain collector, shovel, top soil, manure, compost bin, and seeds

Gather herb plants and seeds

Think of your purpose, unique flavor, and companion planting when choosing your herbs

Grow Your Garden

Research how to best care for your plants via soil, sun, and water recommendations

Adjust your strategies based on plant health

Ensure clean water and compost as feed

Deadhead often

Employ natural pesticides, as needed, such as: garlic, coffee grinds, chili pepper, and tomato leaf spray

Appreciate and watch your plants grow!

Harvesting

Make sure to pick in a V fashion so that the top growers continue to thrive.

Do not over harvest

Creating herbalism goodies

Gather menstruums- 80+ proof alcohol, vinegar,
clean water, carrier oils

Gather tools- tincture droppers, paper bags, mason
jars, muslin cloth, natural twine

Pair based on tastes and actions

Sustainability

Utilize the principles of biodynamics and
permaculture

Safe and ethical wildcrafting

Consult end of year checklist for garden

Heather's Tips for beginning an Herbal Journey:

Be creative, explore new tastes, and new ways of
connecting with the earth

Expand your vision on what health and holism truly
means- once you expand yourself, I guarantee

herbalism will open and reveal more about yourself and the earth than you ever thought possible

Do your research on how to work with herbs you are interested in

Trial and error is the best way to get your herbal technique finetuned

I encourage you to get to know native plants in your area, but explore other culture's traditional medicine-making, too!

Bibliography:

1. Marshall, Michael. "Timeline: The Evolution of Life." New Scientist, www.newscientist.com/article/dn17453-timeline-the-evolution-of-life/.

2. Petrovska, Biljana Bauer. "Historical Review of Medicinal Plants' Usage." Pharmacognosy Reviews, Medknow Publications & Media Pvt Ltd, 2012, www.ncbi.nlm.nih.gov/pmc/articles/PMC3358962/.

3. "Most-Read Articles during April 2019 -- Updated Monthly." Reports - Most-Read Articles during April 2019 -- Updated Monthly, iv.iiarjournals.org/reports/most-read.

4. "Herbal History." Herbal Academy, theherbalacademy.com/herbal-history/.

5. "EWG." EWG, www.ewg.org/.

6. Claudio, Luz. "Planting Healthier Indoor Air." Environmental Health Perspectives, National Institute of Environmental Health Sciences, Oct. 2011, www.ncbi.nlm.nih.gov/pmc/articles/PMC3230460/.

7. Whitaker, Alex. "Herbalism ." Herb-Lore (Herbalism)., www.ancient-wisdom.com/herblore.htm.

8. "Traditional Chinese Medicine: What You Need To Know." National Center for Complementary and Integrative Health, U.S. Department of Health and Human Services, 29 Apr. 2019,

nccih.nih.gov/health/whatiscam/chinesemed.h
tm.

9. "Ayurveda | Ministry of AYUSH | आयुष मंत्रालय |
   GoI." Ministry of AYUSH | GOI,
   ayush.gov.in/about-the-systems/ayurveda.

10. Koithan, Mary, and Cynthia Farrell.
    "Indigenous Native American Healing
    Traditions." The Journal for Nurse
    Practitioners : JNP, U.S. National Library of
    Medicine, 1 June 2010,
    www.ncbi.nlm.nih.gov/pmc/articles/PMC2913
    884/.

11. Zmark.net, Zmark Software design.
    "Echinacea." Herbal Medicine: Echinacea From
    Native American Panacea to Modern
    Phytopharmaceutical,
    www.healthy.net/Health/Article/Echinacea_Fr
    om_Native_American_Panacea_to_Modern_
    Phytopharmaceutical/873.

12. Parsons, M, et al. "Raspberry Leaf and Its
    Effect on Labour: Safety and Efficacy."
    Australian College of Midwives Incorporated
    Journal, U.S. National Library of Medicine,
    Sept. 1999,
    www.ncbi.nlm.nih.gov/pubmed/10754818.

13. "Lemon Balm: Revered by Herbalists from
    Ancient Monasteries to Modern Kitchens."
    Vitality Magazine,
    vitalitymagazine.com/article/lemon-balm1/.

14. Renee, Cmok. "Everything You Ever Wanted To
    Know About Rosemary." Foodal, 17 May 2019,
    foodal.com/knowledge/herbs-

spices/everything-you-ever-wanted-to-know-about-rosemary/.

15. Pöldinger, W. "History of St. Johns Wort." Praxis, U.S. National Library of Medicine, 14 Dec. 2000, www.ncbi.nlm.nih.gov/pubmed/11155493.

16. "Healthy Pregnancy for Mum and Bub." Mr Vitamins News, 8 Mar. 2019, www.mrvitamins.com.au/news/womens-health/natural-fertility-and-pregnancy/healthy-pregnancy/.

17. Stobart, Anne. "The Working of Herbs, Part 5: Medicinal Herb Constituents and Actions." The Recipes Project, recipes.hypotheses.org/3076.

18. "Plant Hardiness." http://tcpermaculture.blogspot.com/2012/01/plant-hardiness-zones-maps-for-world.html

About the Expert

Heather got her Masters in Public Health, majoring in Epidemiology and Global Health in 2017. She has been interested in plant medicine her whole life, which only intensified the more she traveled the globe. She is a self- taught herbalist who never stops learning about new herbal usages. She creates all her own beauty and skin products. At any time of the day a "Wild Heather" can been seen in her natural habitat, foraging for herbs. She believes the human potential can sky-rocket with the infinite benefits of working with herbs. Heather uses herbalism to aid in holistic health and treat acute illnesses. She is an avid yogi and travel adventurer. She believes herbs aided her endurance to run marathons, play volleyball, and run Division 1 cross country, all while going to University. Her all-time favorite herbs to work with is yarrow, chamomile, mint, and lavender.

HowExpert publishes quick 'how to' guides on all topics from A to Z by everyday experts. Visit HowExpert.com to learn more.

Recommended Resources

- <u>HowExpert.com</u> – Quick 'How To' Guides on All Topics by Everyday Experts.
- <u>HowExpert.com/books</u> – HowExpert Books
- <u>HowExpert.com/products</u> – HowExpert Products
- <u>HowExpert.com/courses</u> – HowExpert Courses
- <u>HowExpert.com/clothing</u> – HowExpert Clothing
- <u>HowExpert.com/membership</u> – Learn All Topics from A to Z by Real Experts.
- <u>HowExpert.com/affiliates</u> – HowExpert Affiliate Program
- <u>HowExpert.com/jobs</u> – HowExpert Jobs
- <u>HowExpert.com/writers</u> – Write About Your #1 Passion/Knowledge/Expertise.
- <u>YouTube.com/HowExpert</u> – Subscribe to HowExpert YouTube.
- <u>Instagram.com/HowExpert</u> – Follow HowExpert on Instagram.
- <u>Facebook.com/HowExpert</u> – Follow HowExpert on Facebook.

Printed in Poland
by Amazon Fulfillment
Poland Sp. z o.o., Wrocław

54065665R00045